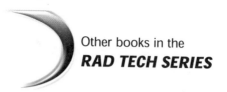

Other books in the
RAD TECH SERIES

Rad Tech's Guide to

Radiation Protection

Euclid Seeram, RTR, BSc, MSc, FCAMRT

Medical Imaging—Advanced Studies
British Columbia Institute of Technology
Burnaby, British Columbia
Canada

b

**Blackwell
Science**

©2001 by Blackwell Science, Inc.

EDITORIAL OFFICES:
Commerce Place, 350 Main Street, Malden, Massachusetts 02148, USA
Osney Mead, Oxford OX2 0EL, England
25 John Street, London WC1N 2BL, England
23 Ainslie Place, Edinburgh EH3 6AJ, Scotland
54 University Street, Carlton, Victoria 3053, Australia

OTHER EDITORIAL OFFICES:
Blackwell Wissenschafts-Verlag GmbH, Kurfürstendamm 57, 10707 Berlin, Germany
Blackwell Science KK, MG Kodenmacho Building, 7-10 Kodenmacho Nihombashi,
    Chuo-ku, Tokyo 104, Japan
Iowa State University Press, A Blackwell Science Company, 2121 S. State Avenue,
    Ames, Iowa 50014-8300, USA

DISTRIBUTORS:
USA
  Blackwell Science, Inc.
  Commerce Place
  350 Main Street
  Malden, Massachusetts 02148
  Telephone orders: (800) 215-1000
    or (781) 388-8250;
  Fax orders: (781) 388-8270
Canada
  Login Brothers Book Company
  324 Saulteaux Crescent
  Winnipeg, Manitoba R3J 3T2
  Telephone orders: (204) 837-2987

Australia
  Blackwell Science Pty, Ltd.
  54 University Street
  Carlton, Victoria 3053
  Telephone orders: 03-9347-0300
  Fax orders: 03-9349-3016
Outside North America and Australia
  Blackwell Science, Ltd.
  c/o Marston Book Services, Ltd.
  P.O. Box 269
  Abingdon
  Oxon OX14 4YN
  England
  Telephone orders: 44-01235-465500
  Fax orders: 44-01235-465555

Acquisitions: Beverly Copland
Development: Julia Casson
Production: GraphCom Corporation
Manufacturing: Lisa Flanagan
Marketing Manager: Toni Fournier
Cover and interior design: Dana Peick, GraphCom Corporation
Typesetting: GraphCom Corporation
Printed and bound by Western Press

Printed in the United States of America
01 02 03 04 5 4 3 2 1

Library of Congress Cataloging-in-Publication Data

Seeram, Euclid.
    Rad tech's guide to radiation protection / by Euclid Seeram.
      p. ; cm.
    Includes bibliographical references and index.
    ISBN 0-86542-580-9
    1. Radiography, Medical—Safety measures. 2. Radiologic technologists—
Health and hygiene.
RC78.3.S437 2001
616.07'57'0289—dc21

                                                            2001025011

This book is dedicated with love and affection to my son, David, a smart, hard-working, caring, and loving individual, and one of my life's treasures.

TABLE OF CONTENTS

PREFACE

Radiation protection is an essential core subject of radiologic technology programs. To meet the needs of these programs, a handful of books on radiation protection is currently available to enable students and technologists alike to acquire the skills required to protect patients, personnel, and members of the public in the radiology department.

In the changing health care environment and, in particular, in the evolution and development of varying degrees of occupational restructuring, there is a need to maintain and enhance technologist competency in a wide variety of areas. *Rad Tech's Guide to Radiation Protection* addresses this need by providing a comprehensive practical guide for technologists engaged in the art and science of radiation protection. An equally important consideration is the need for a single volume that provides students in training with a brief, clear, and concise coverage of the subject in preparation for their professional certification examination.

Rad Tech's Guide to Radiation Protection is not a textbook, and it is not intended to replace the vast resources on radiation protection. Rather, it provides a precis of the extensive coverage of radiation protection topics for technologists.

Rad Tech's Guide to Radiation Protection contains 9 short chapters that cover a wide scope of topics on radiation protection. Chapter 1 discusses the nature and scope of radiation protection and sets the framework for the remaining chapters. Whereas Chapter 2 presents a description of the essential physics for radiation protection, Chapter 3 describes radiation quantities and their units. Chapter 4 outlines the basic concepts of radiobiology and Chapter 5 provides a rationale for radiation protection. Chapters 6 and 7 address the factors that affect dose levels in radiography and fluoroscopy, respectively. Additionally, Chapter 8 provides a discussion of the techniques used to protect individuals from unnecessary radiation exposure. Finally, Chapter 9 reviews radiation protection considerations in pregnancy.

Enjoy the pages that follow and remember—your patients will benefit from your wisdom.

Euclid Seeram, RTR, BSc, MSc, FCAMRT
British Columbia, Canada

ACKNOWLEDGMENTS

Writing a technologist guide such as this one demands a great deal of understanding of the wide and varied resources currently available in the literature, as well as a perception of the contributions of the experts in the fields of radiobiology and radiation protection.

First, I must acknowledge Chris Davis, Executive Editor, who worked at Blackwell Science and who conceived the *Rad Tech Series* idea. Thanks, Chris, for selecting me as "the man for this project" and for all your warm support throughout the years. In addition, Julia Casson, Developmental Editor at Blackwell Science, kept me on track throughout the project. Thanks, Julia. I appreciate your efforts.

I am indeed grateful to all those who have dedicated their energies in providing several comprehensive volumes on medical radiation protection for the radiologic community. First, I would like to acknowledge the notable medical physicist, Dr. Stewart Bushong, and experimental radiobiologist, Dr. Elizabeth Travis. I have learned a great deal on radiologic science from the works of Dr. Bushong, a professor of radiologic science in the Department of Radiology, Baylor College of Medicine, Houston, Texas. In addition, I have gained further insight into the nature, scope, and depth of radiobiology and particularly its significance in radiology, from Dr. Travis, a researcher in the Department of Experimental Radiotherapy, University of Texas, MD Anderson Cancer Center, Houston, Texas.

To all others, such as the authors whose papers I have cited and referenced in this book, thank you for your significant contributions to the radiation protection knowledge base. Additionally, I would like to express my sincere thanks to the publishers of these resources for their permission to reproduce relevant materials from their copyrighted works.

I am also grateful to Dana Peick and her production team at GraphCom Corporation. Thanks for your excellent work.

Finally, I must acknowledge the warm and wonderful support of my family, my lovely wife, Trish, a very caring person, and my handsome son, David, a very special young man; thanks for your love. You both are indeed two of my life's treasures.

Last, but not least, I want to express my gratitude to all the students in my radiation protection classes—your questions have provided me with a further insight into teaching these important subjects.

—ES

CHAPTER 1

Nature and Scope of Radiation Protection

Chapter at a glance

Radiation protection is one of the most important subjects in the education and practice of radiology, because it deals with the safe use of radiation when imaging patients for the purpose of restoring their health.

The purpose of this chapter is to orient the technologist to the nature and scope of radiation protection in diagnostic radiology and to provide a brief overview of topics essential to the theory and practice of radiologic technology.

WHAT IS RADIATION PROTECTION?

Radiation protection is concerned with the protection of persons from the harmful effects of radiation exposure. In diagnostic radiology specifically, radiation protection deals with the protection of both patients and operators, as well as members of the public. Why?

- Patients are exposed to varying amounts of radiation from the x-ray tube, depending on the type of examination.
- Personnel may be exposed to radiation scattered from the patient and the equipment.
- Members of the public are individuals who are working or waiting in close proximity to an x-ray room. These include, for example, secretaries and family members of patients.

SCOPE OF RADIATION PROTECTION

The scope of radiation protection includes knowledge and understanding of the following:

- *Physical factors.* Physical factors are related to the physics of radiation, including energy dissipation in matter, characteristics of radiation, interaction of radiation with matter, and the physical and chemical factors of radiation.
- *Technical factors.* Technical factors include a range of topics such as technical components of imaging systems that affect dose, standards of radiation protection, dose management techniques, and shielding considerations.
- *Procedural factors.* Procedural factors relate to personnel practices during the examination and include such tasks as equipment set-up, patient communication and positioning, selection of technical factors, gonadal shielding, image processing, and image assessment.
- *Biologic factors.* Biologic effects of radiation result from the physical and chemical interaction of radiation with matter (tissue). Bioeffects can be somatic (effects that appear in the individual exposed to radiation) or they can be genetic (effects that appear in the offspring of the individual exposed). Bioeffects can also be classified as stochastic and deterministic (nonstochastic). These are described further in Chapter 3.

Why Protect Patients and Personnel in Radiology?

There are several major reasons for protecting patients undergoing radiologic examinations, as well as personnel conducting the examination. These reasons include:

- Biologic effects data demonstrate beyond question that radiation exposure is harmful to humans.
- Patients receive more radiation exposure from diagnostic radiology compared with any other man-made radiation sources.
- No dose of radiation is considered safe (there is no risk-free dose of radiation).
- Various research studies reveal that some radiologic examinations, particularly involving fluoroscopy and computed tomography, deliver high doses of radiation to patients.
- The technologist assumes full responsibility for all aspects of the radiographic examination, including radiation exposure of the patient. Protection of patients and operators (technologists and radiologists) depends on the technical expertise of both the technologist and the radiologist.
- Radiation safety is required by regulatory authority (United States Center for Devices and Radiological Health [CDRH] under the Food and Drug Administration [FDA], for example, for occupational safety, setting standards for new equipment, and keeping all exposures as low as reasonable achievable [ALARA]).

Framework for Radiation Protection

A *framework* refers to a supporting structure or a basic system. A *radiation protection framework* includes a number of concepts intended to prevent and minimize the harmful effects of radiation exposure.

The International Commission on Radiological Protection (ICRP) offers one comprehensive framework that is accepted by various national radiation protection organizations, including the National Council of Radiation Protection and Measurements (NCRP) in the United States and the Radiation Protection Bureau (RPB) in Canada.

The ICRP framework encompasses several notable concepts, including the types of exposure from which individuals can receive radiation doses and a concept of significance to technologists and radiologists called the two triads of radiation protection.

The types of exposure include:

- *Occupational exposure.* Exposure from work activities.
- *Medical exposure.* Exposure from diagnostic and therapy procedures, which does not include occupational exposure.
- *Public exposure.* All other exposures from natural sources of radiation, such as radon gas.

There are several other concepts that constitute the ICRP framework. However, the two triads of radiation protection will be discussed here. These two triads define current radiation protection standards and include:

- Radiation protection principles
- Radiation protection actions

Radiation Protection Principles

Radiation protection principles include the following three fundamental guiding concepts:

- *Justification.* This concept focuses on net benefit. That is, there must be a benefit associated with any new modality, procedure, or exposure.
- *Optimization.* This concept dictates that all exposures be kept as low as reasonable achievable (ALARA), taking into consideration social and economic factors.
- *Dose limitation.* By establishing dose limits to persons exposed to radiation, certain harmful effects can be prevented and others can be minimized. These limits are numerical values representing an upper limit of exposure annually. For example, the annual dose limit to the lens of the eye is 150 millisieverts (mSv) or 15,000 millirem (mrem) for occupationally exposed individuals. The annual whole-body occupational dose limit (technologists) is 50 mSv (5000 mrem).

Dose limits are discussed in a later chapter of this book.

Radiation Protection Actions

Radiation protections actions are based on the following three concepts:

- **Time.** Because dose is directionally proportional to the length of time of the exposure, it is important to decrease the time of the exposure to decrease the dose. If the time is decreased by a factor of two, then the dose will be reduced by a factor of two.
- **Shielding.** To reduce the dose to patients and others, it is essential to place a shield between the source of radiation (x-ray tube) and the individual exposed (patient). Gonadal shielding is a prime example of this concept.
- **Distance.** The dose an individual receives is inversely proportional to the square of the distance. This factor is known as the inverse square law and it is expressed as

$$I = 1/d^2$$

where I equals intensity of the radiation and d equals the distance from the source of the radiation to the individual exposed. As the distance is increased, the dose is reduced proportionally to the square of the distance.

BASIC SCHEMES FOR PATIENT EXPOSURE IN RADIOGRAPHY AND FLUOROSCOPY

The basic scheme for patient exposure refers to the beam geometry used to expose the anatomic area of interest. The beam geometry refers to the size and shape of the x-ray beam emanating from the x-ray tube. Beam geometry also refers to whether the beam is fixed or is moving during the exposure.

Radiography

In radiography:

- The beam geometry describes an open beam shaped by the collimator to fall on the area of interest on the patient.
- The beam is fixed on this area of interest during the exposure.
- The beam is collimated to the size of the image receptor (film cassette) used for the examination.

- Radiographic exposure technique factors, such as mA, kVp, and exposure time in seconds, are used to produce images.
- Images are static and each image requires a separate exposure.

Fluoroscopy
In fluoroscopy:
- The beam geometry describes an open beam shaped by the collimator to fall on the regions of interest being imaged.
- The beam is moving during fluoroscopic exposures. This movement is necessary to track the flow of contrast media through the anatomy, such as the gastrointestinal tract.
- The beam is collimated to the size of the image receptor using cassette-loaded spot films.
- Fluoroscopic exposure technique factors (generally low mA [approximately 1 to 3 mA] and high kVp) are used to show fluoroscopic images displayed on a television monitor. The x-ray tube is energized for longer periods compared with the short exposure times used in radiography.
- Radiographic exposure technique factors are used for cassette-loaded spot films recorded by the radiologist during the examination and by the technologist who records "overhead" images after the fluoroscopic portion of the examination. This is the radiographic component of a routine fluoroscopic examination.

FACTORS AFFECTING DOSE IN DIAGNOSTIC RADIOLOGY

To protect patients, personnel, and members of the public from radiation in diagnostic radiology, it is mandatory that technologists have a firm understanding of the various factors affecting dose. In this text, only dose factors in radiography and fluoroscopy will be considered.

Radiographic Factors
The technical factors affecting patient dose in radiography are:
- Type of x-ray generator
- X-ray exposure technique factors (mA, kVp, and time)

- Beam energy and filtration
- Collimation and field size
- Distance from the x-ray tube to the patient (source-to-skin distance) and the distance from the x-ray tube to the image receptor (SID)
- Patient thickness and density
- Antiscatter grids
- Image receptor sensitivity
- Film processing
- Shielding
- Repeat examinations
- Patient orientation

Fluoroscopic Factors

The technical factors affecting dose in fluoroscopy are numerous and include:

- Beam energy and tube current
- Collimation
- Source-to-skin distance
- Patient-to-image intensifier distance
- Beam-on time
- Antiscatter grids
- Image magnification
- Image recording techniques
- Conduct of the fluoroscopic portion of the examination
- Conduct of the radiographic portion of the fluoroscopic examination

These factors are elaborated further in Chapter 6.

DOSE MANAGEMENT TECHNIQUES

The goal of radiation protection is to reduce the dose to patients and personnel. Dose management techniques are intended to optimize the imaging process to produce diagnostic image quality using the ALARA philosophy. These techniques are governed objectively by guidelines and recommendations of not only the ICRP, but also by various national regulatory authorities and by radiation protection organizations issuing Radiation Protection Reports. The guidelines and recommendations for dose management in radiology address the four major areas.

■ *Equipment design and performance.* Equipment must be designed or upgraded to meet certain specifications that will allow the operator to optimize image quality while protecting patients and personnel from unnecessary radiation. These guidelines and recommendations focus on specific technical parameters such as filtration, collimation, and source-to-skin distance for radiographic and fluoroscopic (fixed and mobile) equipment.

■ *Personnel practices.* These recommendations focus on the conduct of the examination using the ALARA philosophy. For example, the primary beam must always be collimated to the size of the image receptor or smaller; technologists should not hold patients to achieve immobilization during an examination.

■ *Shielding.* Shielding is one of three radiation-protection actions intended to protect individuals from radiation exposure. Recommendations for shielding address the use of lead shields to protect radiosensitive organs such as the gonads. Additionally, walls of x-ray rooms are lined with lead to prevent radiation from penetrating and exposing individuals outside the x-ray room.

■ *Education and training.* Guidelines and recommendations for the safe use of radiation also address the need for operators to be educated and trained in a wide range of subjects. These subjects include radiation physics, instrumentation, radiation risks, radiation protection, and are intended to minimize the radiation dose to patients, personnel, and members of the public. These techniques will be described further in Chapter 7.

PREGNANCY: RADIATION PROTECTION CONSIDERATIONS

This is an important topic in radiation protection for everyone working in radiology because of the sensitivity of the conceptus (any product of conception, embryo or fetus) to radiation.

There are several major considerations with respect to in utero exposure in radiology. It is not within the scope of this chapter to outline all of the factors relating to in utero exposure. However, a few significant points to be noted are as follows:

- Data suggest that, depending on the dose and gestational stage of exposure, there can be malformations and radiation-induced childhood malignancy.
- If a patient must have an x-ray examination (because the benefits outweigh the risks), then several precautions should be taken:
    - Shielding must be used only if it will not interfere with diagnostic information.
    - High-kVp techniques and increased filtration are advocated.
    - Fluoroscopy must be kept to an "absolute minimum."
    - The number of films must be kept to a minimum.
- Several factors affect dose to the fetus, including the technical factors previously mentioned. Additionally, direct exposure (fetus in the field-of-view) and indirect exposure (fetus outside the field-of-view) are significant factors.
- Fetal doses can be estimated to provide information on the risks to the fetus and on any actions to be taken.
- Following an exposure, the NCRP (Report 54) recommendations should be observed. These points are examined in chapter 8.
- Ultrasound (rather than radiology) is now used to evaluate fetal maturation and placental localization.

Several issues and concerns surround the pregnant technologist. The pregnant technologist should notify the department of her pregnancy and use a second dosimeter for the remainder of the pregnancy (under the apron at the waist level). The work schedule of a pregnant technologist may be altered.

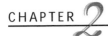

Diagnostic X-Rays:
Physical Factors

Chapter at a glance

X-ray films are produced when high-speed electrons strike a target. In diagnostic radiology, an x-ray tube is used to produce x-ray films for patients. The x-ray tube consists basically of an anode and a cathode. The cathode consists of a filament that when heated emits electrons. In turn, the electrons are accelerated at high speeds to strike a small spot on the anode, called the target. The electron-target interaction results in the production of heat and x-ray films.

The purpose of this chapter is to outline several physical factors relating to the basic physics of x-ray production, x-ray interactions with matter, and x-ray attenuation, all of which are important to radiation protection. An understanding of how the x-ray beam is produced, how it interacts with the patient, and what happens when the beam is transmitted through the patient is key to optimizing image quality and minimizing radiation dose. The technologist has control over several parameters affecting x-ray production, attenuation, and interaction of x-rays with the patient.

This chapter is pivotal in ensuring that the technologist has the fundamental skills for good radiation protection practices.

X-Ray Production

To produce x-ray films for a particular examination, the technologist sets up the appropriate kVp, mA, and time (in seconds) on the control panel. These exposure technique factors determine the type of radiation beam that will be produced by the x-ray tube. In this section, the following points will be summarized: the mechanisms by which electrons from the filament of the x-ray tube create x-ray films; the x-ray emission spectrum, including x-ray quantity, quality, and the factors affecting both; and finally, x-ray attenuation.

Mechanisms for Creating X-Rays

There are two mechanisms by which high-speed electrons from the filament of an x-ray tube create x-rays. There are the characteristic and the bremsstrahlung processes, which give rise to characteristic and bremsstrahlung radiation.

- *Characteristic radiation.* When a high-speed electron from the filament interacts with an inner-shell electron of the target atom, and the electron has enough kinetic energy, then the electron will be ejected from its orbit leaving a vacancy in the orbit. An electron from an outer shell will move into the inner-shell vacancy. This movement results in an emission of characteristic x-rays, as shown in Figure 2-1.

- *Bremsstrahlung radiation.* A result of electrons interacting with the target nucleus rather than the electrons. The production of bremsstrahlung (brems) radiation is illustrated in Figure 2-2. When incident electrons approach the charged nucleus, they decelerate, change direction, and exit with reduced energy. This loss of energy appears in the form of radiation called brems radiation.

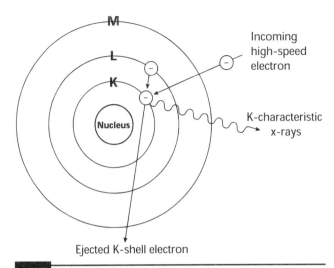

Figure 2-1 Characteristic x rays are emitted when an inner-shell electron is ejected from the atom (ionization) and an outer-shell electron moves in to fill the vacancy in the inner shell. *(Reproduced with permission from Seeram E.* Radiation protection. *Philadelphia: Lippincott, 1997.)*

The following points are important with respect to characteristic and brems radiation in diagnostic radiology:

- In the range of kVp values used in diagnostic radiology for general radiographic and fluoroscopic procedures, most of the x-rays emitted from the tube are brems radiation.
- In mammography, however, characteristic radiation is used since the narrow band of energy is most useful when imaging the soft tissues of the breast.
- K-characteristic radiation is used in radiography.
- Brems radiation has a wide range of energies suitable for all radiography and fluoroscopy examinations.
- The output radiation from the x-ray tube consists of both brems and characteristic radiation. If the intensity of the radiation is plotted as a function of its energy, then an x-ray emission spectrum is the result.

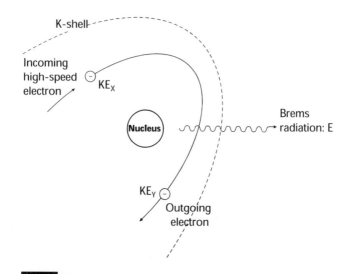

Figure 2-2 Brems radiation is emitted from the x-ray tube when high-speed electrons interact with the nucleus of the target atoms. Electrons slow down, change direction, and leave with reduced kinetic energy. This loss of energy results in brems radiation. *(Reproduced with permission from Seeram E.* Radiation protection. *Philadelphia: Lippincott, 1997.)*

X-RAY SPECTRUM

When a technologist makes an exposure for an examination, both characteristic and brems radiation are emitted from the tube. This emission is known as the emission x-ray spectrum, which is a graph illustrating of the intensity of x-rays (number of x-rays per unit energy) plotted as a function of the x-ray energy.

Form of X-Ray Spectrum:
- The general form of an x-ray emission spectrum is shown in Figure 2-3.
- Two spectra are shown:
    1. Brems or continuous spectrum
    2. Characteristic or discrete spectrum.

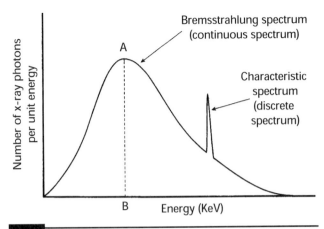

Figure 2-3 The form and shape of the brems and characteristic x-ray spectra. *(Reproduced with permission from
Seeram E. Radiation protection. Philadelphia: Lippincott,
1997.)*

An understanding of both of these spectra helps the technologist realize how exposure technique factors and filtration
can affect image quality and radiation dose.

- The area under the curve represents the number of photons in the x-ray beam. Greater area indicates more
  photons, thus a higher dose. The area is also referred to
  as the x-ray quantity.
- The energy distribution of the beam is shown on the
  horizontal axis and is expressed in keV. The term x-ray
  quality is used to describe the energy distribution, thus
  the shape of the curve.

X-Ray Beam Quality and Quantity

The intensity of the beam from the tube can be described in
terms of both quantity and quality. Quantity and quality of the
beam emanating from the x-ray tube affect the dose to the
patient.

- *X-ray quantity,* also referred to as radiation exposure,
  refers to the number of photons in the beam. More photons increase the dose to the patient. Numerous factors
  determine x-ray quantity.

- *X-ray quality* refers to the energy or penetrating power of the photons in the beam. The beam consists of both high-energy and low-energy photons. Numerous factors affect beam quality.

Controlling Beam Quality and Quantity

There are several factors affecting the quality and quantity of the x-ray beam. However, few are under the direct control of the technologist.

The factors affecting quality and quantity are:

- *kVp.* kVp is under the direct control of the technologist. The penetration of the beam and the beam quality is greater as the kVp increases. High-kVp techniques result in a low dose. The beam intensity is directly proportional to the kVp^2. If the kVp is doubled, then the intensity increases by a factor of four. This factor means that by increasing the kVp, the quantity can be increased. Increasing the kVp by 15% is comparable to doubling the mAs.

- *mA/mAs.* mA/mAs is under the direct control of the technologist. mA/mAs affects the quantity of radiation in that the quantity is proportional to the mA. If the mA is doubled, then the quantity is doubled, and the dose is increased by a factor of two. The same applies to the mAs.

- *Filtration.* Filtration affects both the quality and quantity of the beam. A filter is always inserted in the x-ray beam to remove low-energy photons. This removal reduces the quantity, and as a result, the mean energy of the beam increases. The beam becomes more penetrating or harder. Thicker filters reduce the quantity of the beam, but increases beam quality. A filter is intended to protect the patient by removing these low-energy photons.

- *Target material.* Target materials with higher atomic numbers increase both the quantity of photons slightly and the quality (energy) of the beam. Tungsten produces a significantly more efficient spectrum than molybdenum. The technologist has no control over this parameter.

■ *Type of generator.* The x-ray generator provides power to energize the x-ray tube to produce x-rays. This generator determines the voltage waveform to the tube. Three types of generators are available: single-phase, three-phase, and high-frequency generators. State-of-the-art x-ray equipment use high-frequency generators, which are more efficient since they produce greater quantity of photons (area under the curve) with higher effective energies (greater quality) than single- and three-phase generators. This means that the dose can be reduced using high-frequency generators by appropriately adjusting exposure technique factors (e.g., high-kVp techniques can be used).

■ *Source-to-image receptor distance (SID).* The SID is under the direct control of the technologist. The SID affects the quantity of photons but has no effect on the quality. The quantity is affected by the inverse square law, which states that the intensity (quantity) is inversely proportional to the square of the distance. If the distance is increased, then the quantity decreases by $1/d^2$.

In summary, the effect of various equipment parameters on x-ray quantity and quality is shown in Table 2-1.

X-Ray Attenuation

Definition

When a beam of x-rays pass through matter, it is attenuated before it reaches the image receptor (Figure 2-4).

■ *Attenuation* is the reduction in the intensity of the beam as it passes through any material.

■ The materials that are of importance in radiology are, of course, the x-ray tube filter and the patient.

■ The reduction in intensity is a result of absorption and deflection of photons from the radiation beam.

■ Absorption of photons produces a greater dose to the patient.

■ Increased attenuation produces more absorption, thus increasing the dose to the patient.

TABLE 2-1	Effects of Various Parameters on Quality and Quantity of X Rays	
VARIABLE	QUANTITY	QUALITY
Anode material (Z)	$\alpha\ Z$	Affects position (energy) of characteristic x rays
Tube potential (kVp)	$\alpha\ kVp^2$	Determines presence or absence of characteristic x rays; determines maximum x-ray energy
Tube current (mA)	$\alpha\ mA$	None
Time	α time	None
Distance	$\alpha\ 1/distance^2$	None
Filtration (HVL)	Decreases with increasing filtration (higher HVL)	Increased percentage of high-energy x rays with increased filtration (higher HVL)
Waveform	Increases with decreasing voltage ripple (flatter waveform)	Increased percentage of high-energy x rays with decreased filtration (flatter waveform)

From McCollough CH. X-Ray production. Radiographics 1997;18:967–984. Reproduced with permission.

- A measure of the radiation quantity attenuated by a given thickness of material is defined as the attenuation coefficient.
- The linear attenuation coefficient (μ) is the fractional reduction of the radiation per-unit thickness of the material traversed.
- Although μ is a measure of per unit length attenuation, it can also be expressed as per unit mass of the absorbing material. This is the mass attenuation coefficient, which is equal to μ divided by the density (ρ) of the material. The unit of μ/ρ is centimeter^2 per gram (cm^2/g).
- The attenuation of a monoenergetic beam (all photons have the same energy or are monochromatic) of x-rays or gamma rays is shown in Figure 2-5. The following points are important:
  - Equal thicknesses of absorber remove equal amounts of radiation

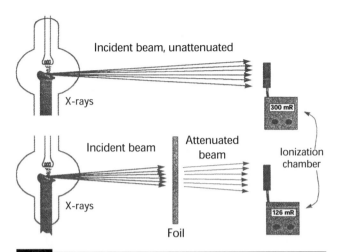

Figure 2-4 Attenuation is the reduction of the intensity of an x-ray beam as it passes through any material. *(Reproduced with permission from McKetty MH. X-ray attenuation.* Radiographics *1998;18:151–163.)*

❏ The attenuation is exponential, as shown in the following graph and described by the equation:

$$N = N_0\, e^{-\mu x}$$

where N_0 = number of incident photon
N = number of transmitted photons
e = base of the natural logarithm
x = thickness of the material

❏ Additionally, the attenuation can be described by the equation:

$$I = I_0\, e^{-\mu x}$$

where I_0 = intensity of the incident photons
I = intensity of the transmitted photons
e = base of the natural logarithm
x = thickness of the material

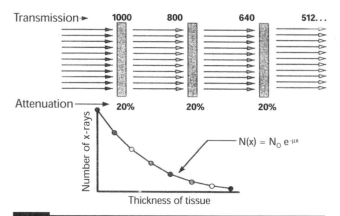

Figure 2-5 Exponential attenuation of a homogeneous (monochromatic) beam of radiation in which all the photons have the same energy. *(Reproduced by permission from McKetty MH. X-ray attenuation.* Radiographics *1998;18:151-163.)*

- The x-ray beam from the x-ray tube is a heterogeneous or polychromatic beam in which the photons have different energies, and the attenuation is somewhat different from a monochromatic or homogeneous beam.
- The attenuation of a heterogeneous beam is illustrated in Figure 2-6. The following points are important:
- Equal thicknesses of material remove different amounts of radiation.
  - ❑ Low-energy photons are attenuated more rapidly compared with high-energy photons. This event changes both the quantity and quality of the beam.
  - ❑ The beam quantity decreases and the beam quality increases. That is, the mean energy of the photons increases. This increase is referred to as beam hardening, a term used to indicate that the beam is more penetrating.

Factors Affecting Attenuation

Since attenuation affects the dose to the patient through the absorption process, it is necessary to examine the factors that increase attenuation (more patient dose) and factors that decrease attenuation (less patient dose). These factors include:

Heterogeneous
beam

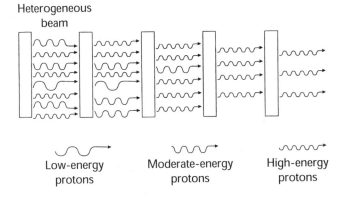

Low-energy
protons

Moderate-energy
protons

High-energy
protons

Figure 2-6 Attenuation of a heterogeneous beam of radiation.
See text for further explanation. *(Reproduced with
permission from Seeram E. Radiation protection.
Philadelphia: Lippincott, 1997.)*

- ■ *Thickness of the absorbing material.* In general, the thicker the material is, the greater the attenuation becomes.
- ■ *Density (mass per unit volume).* As the density of the
  material increases, attenuation increases.
- ■ *Atomic number (Z) or number of protons in the nucleus.* As
  Z increases, attenuation increases. Contrast agents—barium and iodine compounds—increase attenuation.
  Contrast agents are used to visualize blood vessels and
  the gastrointestinal track because their Z are different
  than the surrounding soft tissue. These compounds atten-
  uate more radiation rendering them visible on the film.
- ■ *Beam energy.* This factor is determined by the kVp used
  to image the material (patient).
  - ❑ Low kVp results in more absorption of the beam
    (increased attenuation), thus a higher dose to the
    patient.
  - ❑ High kVp results in more transmission of the beam
    through the patient (less absorption), thus a lesser
    dose to the patient.

To understand how beam energy and attenuation are related, it is necessary to explain what occurs when x-rays interact
with matter.

X-RAY INTERACTIONS

One of the goals of radiology is to optimize image quality while reducing the dose to the patient. It is the nature of the interactions of radiation with matter that determines not only image contrast, but also the dose to the patient.

There are several interactions of radiation with matter, including Rayleigh (coherent) scattering, photoelectric absorption, Compton scattering, and pair production. Among these, the photoelectric absorption and Compton scattering are the most important attenuation mechanisms in diagnostic radiology. Therefore only these two will be presented in this chapter. The others do not occur with any noticeable significance in diagnostic radiology. The physics of the interactions will not be described, but rather, a basic overview will be presented to demonstrate how these two interactions relate to dose to the patient, as well as beam energy.

Photoelectric Absorption

The photoelectric absorption (also referred to as the photoelectric effect) is shown in Figure 2-7. The following points are noteworthy:

- The incident photon interacts with an inner-shell (K or L) electron (tightly bound).
- The photon is completely absorbed and the electron is ejected from the atom. This electron is called a photoelectron.
- The absorption of the incident photons in this interaction increases the dose to the patient since they do not pass through the patient and reach the image receptor.
- The probability that the photoelectric effect will occur depends on the photon energy (E) and the atomic number (Z) of the absorbing material.
- The probability is directly proportional to Z^3 and inversely proportional to E^3.
- At low beam energies (low-kVp techniques) the photoelectric effect predominates and the patient dose increases. However, image contrast is greater in materials with high Z.

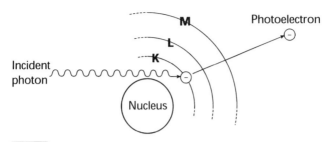

Figure 2-7 Photoelectric absorption is an attenuation mechanism whereby an incident photon interacts with inner-shell electrons, ejecting them from the atom. See text for further explanation. *(Reproduced with permission from Seeram E.* Radiation protection. *Philadelphia: Lippincott, 1997.)*

Compton Scattering

Another x-ray interaction that is significant in diagnostic radiology is Compton scattering, as shown in Figure 2-8. In Compton scattering:

- Incident photons interact with free electrons, which are loosely bound electrons in the outer shell of the atom.
- The incident photon is scattered in a new direction with energy less than that of the incident photon.
- The incident photon also ejects the electron from its orbit. This electron is called a recoil or scattered electron.
- The scattered photons (scattered radiation) reach the film and degrade image contrast. Compton scattering produces most of the scattered radiation in diagnostic radiology.
- The probability that a Compton interaction will occur depends on the number of outer-shell electrons and the photon energy (E).
- Compton interaction is directly proportional to the number of outer-shell electrons and inversely proportional to E. Characteristics of a Compton interaction are:
  - As the number of outer-shell electrons (loosely bound electrons) increases, Compton scattering increases.

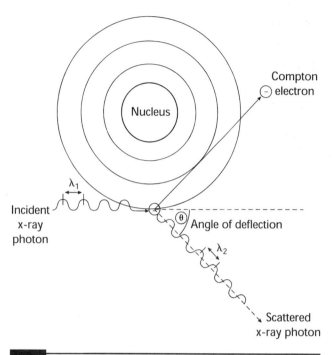

Figure 2-8 Compton interaction or scattering is an attenuation mechanism whereby an incident photon interacts with an outer-shell electron and ejects it from the atom. The incident photon loses its energy and changes direction of travel. This deflected photon is the scattered photon that may reach the film and destroy image contrast. *(Reproduced with permission from Seeram E. Radiation protection. Philadelphia: Lippincott, 1997.)*

❏ As the x-ray energy increases, the probability of Compton interaction decreases.

❏ The probability of Compton interaction relative to photoelectric absorption increases.

❏ The probability of penetration of the beam through the absorber without interaction increases.

■ In radiography and fluoroscopy, the patient is the major source of scattered radiation. Technologists and radiologists must protect themselves from exposure to scatter by remaining in the control booth or by wearing protective aprons during the exposure.

INCREASING kVp AND SCATTER PRODUCTION

High-kVp techniques are used in diagnostic radiology to penetrate the anatomy (as well as contrast agents such as barium) and to reduce the dose to the patient. High-kVp techniques produce films with poor image contrast resulting from the increasing scatter that reaches the film. This effect is explained by Dendy and Heator.

- Scatter production in the patient is decreased because the probability of Compton interaction decreases with increasing kVp. "A smaller amount of primary radiation is required to produce a given density on the film as film density is proportional to kVp^4."
- The forward scatter leaving the patient and reaching the film increases because:
    - The fraction of the total scatter produced, traveling in a forward direction, increases as the kVp rises.
    - The mean energy of the scattered radiation increases, thus less of it is absorbed by the patient.

Therefore the major reason for an increase in scatter at the film is the increase in the mean energy of the scatter.

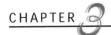

Radiation Quantities and Units

Chapter at a glance

Human beings are exposed to several sources of radiation and are subject to different types of radiation exposure. Quantifying ionizing radiation and biologic risks demands an understanding of radiation quantities and the units associated with each of them.

The purpose of this chapter is to identify two major sources of radiation exposure and define the situations in which individuals are exposed to radiation. In addition, several radiation quantities and their units will be highlighted.

These topics are important to the technologist for several reasons:

- Annual dose limits for individuals are based on the types of exposure.
- Dose magnitudes from various radiological procedures are often compared with those from natural background radiation exposure.
- Dose limits demand a clear understanding of radiation quantities and their associated units.
- Radiation quantities and their units are essential ingredients when quantifying ionizing radiation and biologic risks.
- Measuring and reporting patient dose in radiology require the intelligent use of these quantities.

SOURCES OF RADIATION EXPOSURE

There are two main sources of radiation exposure:

- Natural radiation sources
- Man-made radiation sources

Natural radiation sources are composed of three major categories: cosmic radiation, earth sources (terrestrial radiation), and internal sources.

- Among the natural sources, radon contributes the highest exposure to the population. Specifically, radon-222 (^{222}Rn) is a naturally occurring radioactive gas that arises from the radioactive decay of radium-226 (^{226}Ra). Radon exposure is particularly important to the public since its intensity depends on where an individual lives. Radon gas can enter a building. Breathing radon gas can expose the lungs to alpha particles, which the gas emits. When the level of radon gas exceeds 4 picocuries per liter (pCi/L) in a building, the United States Environmental Protection Agency (EPA) recommends that efforts be made to eliminate or reduce this exposure.
- Cosmic radiation includes solar (e.g., protons, helium) and galactic radiation (e.g., gamma rays, high-energy protons, neutrons). Cosmic radiation intensity depends on latitude and altitude and is greatest at the poles and is

less at the equator. Additionally, cosmic radiation increases with altitude.

■ Earth sources include radiation from the air, terrestrial radiation, radiation from buildings, and endogenous radiation. The last source refers to radiation arising from several internal body sources, such as carbon-14, potassium-40, rubidium-87, and strontium-90. Sleeping with a partner will increase an individual's exposure.

Man-made radiation sources, conversely, consist of several sources, including medical x-rays, nuclear medicine, consumer products (e.g., smoke alarms), and other sources such as fallout from nuclear testing.

■ Medical x-ray exposure represents the greatest source of exposure to the population.

■ Nuclear medicine examinations result in the second largest man-made radiation source compared with all others.

Exposures from medical x-rays and nuclear medicine procedures constitute medical exposure, compared with other types of exposure such as occupational exposure and public exposure.

TYPES OF EXPOSURES

The International Commission on Radiological Protection (ICRP) identifies three situations in which individuals are exposed to radiation. These situations include:

Occupational Exposure
This situation refers to all exposures received in the workplace by radiologic technologists. All exposures received when working in radiography, fluoroscopy, mobile and operating room radiography, computed tomography, and angiography constitute occupational exposure. Occupational exposure excludes medical exposure.

Medical Exposure
This situation includes exposures from medical and therapy procedures for diagnosis and treatment, respectively. It also includes exposures resulting from individuals assisting patients having diagnostic or therapeutic examinations. It does not include radiation scattered from patients having examinations or occupational exposure of staff members.

Public Exposure

The ICRP states that:

> "Public exposure encompasses all exposures other than occupational and medical exposures. The component of public exposure due to natural sources is by far the largest, but this provides no justification for reducing the attention paid to smaller but more readily controlled exposures to artificial sources" (p. 34).

QUANTITIES AND UNITS FOR QUANTIFYING IONIZING RADIATION

In Figure 3-1, three radiation quantities and their associated units are shown. Two of them—exposure and absorbed dose—refer to the radiation; the third—dose equivalent—relates to the biologic risk of the radiation absorption. In this section, we focus only on quantities and units for quantifying ionizing radiation.

Recently, the ICRP began using the International System of Units (SI units) for radiation quantities. SI units are now used in several countries, including Canada. In the United States, the NCRP made the following statement with respect to the use of SI units in radiation protection and measurements: "After 1989, it is recommended that SI units be used exclusively. In tables, graphs, and radiation records, one system of units would be used with a footnote containing conversion factors to the other system" (p. 2).

SI units are used throughout this book.

Exposure

Exposure is a radiation quantity referring to the intensity of radiation. Exposure:

- Can be measured using an ionization chamber, which contains a volume of air.
- Ionizes the air in the chamber.
- Is the total change liberated in a cubic centimeter of air.
- Is measured in coulombs per kilogram (C/kg) in the SI system and in roentgens (R) in the old system of units.
- Of $1 R = 2.58 \times 10^{-4}$ C/kg; $1 C = 1.6 \times 10^{19}$ electrons.
- Follows the inverse square law, which states that the intensity of radiation decreases inversely as the square

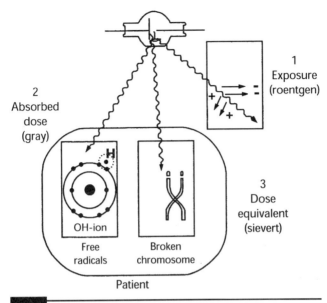

Figure 3-1 Three radiation quantities and their associated units. See text for further explanation. *(Reproduced with permission from Huda W, Slone R. Review of radiologic physics. Baltimore: Williams & Wilkins, 1995.)*

of the distance. If distance from the source of exposure is increased by a factor of three, then the exposure is decreased by a factor of nine:

■ Is equal to the exposure rate multiplied by time. The exposure rate is the exposure per unit time.

KERMA

KERMA is a quantity that characterizes the radiation field.

■ KERMA is an acronym for kinetic energy released per unit mass.

■ KERMA quantifies the energy transferred from the radiation beam to charged particles (protons and electrons) in matter.

■ The unit of KERMA is joules per kilogram (J/kg).

■ KERMA may replace the quantity exposure in the SI system.

Absorbed Dose

Absorbed dose is another quantity to quantify ionizing radiation.

- ■ Absorbed dose (D) is the energy deposited in an absorbing medium from ionizing radiation. (Absorbed dose measures the amount of energy absorbed.)
- ■ The SI unit for absorbed dose is the gray (Gy); the old unit is the rad (radiation absorbed dose).
- ■ 1 Gy = 100 rad.
- ■ 1 rad = 10 mGy.
- ■ 1 Gy of absorbed dose is equal to 1J of energy deposited per kilogram of absorbing medium.
- ■ Biologic effects are associated with the amount of absorbed dose.

f-Factor

When it is necessary to calculate the absorbed dose (D) given only the exposure (E), the *f-factor* is used.

- ■ $D = f \times E$.
- ■ f converts roentgens to rads.
- ■ For radiology, the f-factor for air and soft tissues is approximately 1, although it ranges from 4 (low energy) to 1 (high energy) for bone.

Linear Energy Transfer

The *linear energy transfer* (LET) is a physical factor quantifying the radiation beam.

- ■ LET is the rate at which the radiation transfers energy to surrounding tissues.
- ■ The unit of LET is kilo electron volt per micrometer (keV/μm).
- ■ The LET for x-rays is 3.0 keV/μm and 100 keV/μm for 5-MeV alpha particles.
- ■ As LET increases, bioeffectiveness increases.

QUANTITIES AND UNITS FOR QUANTIFYING BIOLOGIC RISKS

Radiation absorption in biologic systems can lead to excitation and ionization. Both excitation and ionization lead to the production of free radicals, which subsequently produce biologic damage.

Several quantities used to quantify biologic risks of radiation exposure include dose equivalent, equivalent dose, and effective dose.

Dose Equivalent

The *dose equivalent* (H) is a quantity defined for radiation protection purposes. Since different sources of radiation have different efficiencies in producing biologic damage, a quantity is required to address the differences in bioeffectiveness. The dose equivalent represents this quantity.

- Dose equivalent is equal to the absorbed dose (D) multiplied by a quality factor (Q), which depends on the LET of the radiation.

$$H = DQ$$

- The SI unit of H is the sievert (Sv); the old unit is the rem (rad equivalent man).
- The badges worn by technologists record occupational exposure in millisieverts (mSv).
- The sievert is related to absorbed dose as follows:

Sievert = Gray × Radiation Weighting Factor (W_R)

- 1 Sv = 100 rem
- 1 mSv = 100 mrem
- 10 mSv = 1 rem
- For the sake of simplicity (in radiology),

1 Roentgen = 1 rad = 1 rem

- In the SI system,

$$2.58 \times 10^{-4} \text{ C/kg} = 0.01 \text{ Gy} = 0.01 \text{ Sv}$$

Radiation Weighting Factor

Bioeffects of radiation depend not only on the absorbed dose (D), but also on the type and energy of the radiation.

- Radiation weighting factor (W_R) for x-rays and gamma rays is 1, 5 for high-energy protons, and 20 for alpha particles and fission fragments.

Equivalent Dose

In 1990 the ICRP revised its radiation protection recommendations and the term dose equivalent (H) was replaced by the term *equivalent dose* (H_T). While H is the weighted absorbed dose at a point, H_T is the weighted absorbed dose in tissues or organs.

- $H_T = \Sigma\, W_R \cdot D_{TR}$
- The above is read as the equivalent dose is equal to the sum of the weighted absorbed doses. D_{TR} is the absorbed dose averaged over the tissue or organ, T; for the type of radiation, R.

Effective Dose

The *effective dose* (E) was previously referred to as the effective dose equivalent (H_E).

- E is the equivalent dose weighted for the type of tissue (organ).
- E is used to quantify the different risks from partial body exposure compared with risks from an equivalent whole-body dose.
- $E = \Sigma\, W_T \cdot H_T$, where W_T is the tissue weighting factor.
- The SI unity E is sievert (Sv); the old unit is the rem.
- The dose limits recommended for occupational, public, students in training, and the embryo or fetus are expressed as E.
- The effective dose for an upper gastrointestinal tract examination is 2.45 mSv. This value means that the risk from an upper gastrointestinal tract examination is equivalent to the risk of an exposure dose of 2.45 mSv to the whole body.

Tissue Weighting Factor

Bioeffects depend not only on the absorbed dose and type and energy of the radiation, but also on the type of tissue.

- W_T provides data on the relative contribution of the tissue or organ to the total biologic response from whole-body irradiation.
- The W_T for the gonads, bone marrow, breast, and thyroid, for example, are 0.20, 0.12, 0.05, and 0.05, respectively.

RADIATION MEASUREMENT

There are a number of tools currently available for measuring and monitoring the amount of radiation to an individual. Of relevance to diagnostic radiology include the ionization chamber, film dosimetry, and thermoluminescent dosimetry.

Ionization Chamber
The ionization chamber consists of a gas-filled chamber and is used to measure radiation exposure.

- When radiation falls on the chamber, the gas ionizes to produce ions, which are collected and counted.
- The total charge (Q coulombs) determines the exposure expressed in Roentgens or C/kg.
- Ionization chambers are used as dosimetry devices to measure the output from an x-ray tube. These chambers are also used in automatic exposure timing.
- A pocket ionization chamber can be used for personnel dosimetry (i.e., to measure occupational exposures).

Film Dosimetry
Film dosimetry is used to monitor occupational exposures in the form of a film badge.

- The film badge consists of small x-ray films placed between special filters to detect beta, gamma, and x-rays.
- These badges can detect occupational exposure at or above 0.1 mSv (10 mrem) and are not sensitive to detect lower levels of exposure.
- Film dosimetry is being replaced by thermoluminescent dosimetry.

Thermoluminescent Dosimetry
Thermoluminescent dosimetry (TLD) can be used to measure patient exposures and to monitor personnel occupational exposures.

- TLD is based on thermoluminescence.
- Lithium fluoride (LiF) chips are used in diagnostic radiology.
- When exposed to x-rays, electrons in the LiF are raised to another energy and are trapped there until the TLD

chip is heated. This heating causes the electrons to return to their original orbits causing the emission of light. The amount of light emitted is directly proportional to the radiation exposure.

- TLD can measure doses from 0.1 mGy (10 mrad) to approximately 10 Gy (1000 mrad).

WEARING A PERSONNEL DOSIMETER

In radiography and fluoroscopy, technologists must wear personnel dosimeters to record their occupational exposures in millisieverts.

- In radiography, the dosimeter can be worn at the level of the waist, at the level of the collar in the upper chest area, or on the anterior surface of the individual.
- In fluoroscopy, when a protective apron must be worn, the NCRP (1989) states:

  "When the apron is worn, a decision must be made as to whether to wear one or more than one dosimeter. If only one is worn and it is worn under the apron, it can represent the dose to most internal organs, but it may underestimate the dose to the head and neck (including the thyroid gland). If only one is worn and it is worn at the collar, it may represent the dose to the organs contained in the head and neck, but it may over estimate the dose to the organs in the trunk of the body" (p. 49).

- The Canadian Radiation Safety Code (RPB, 1992) states that for diagnostic radiology, the dosimeter must be worn under the apron; and when the radiation levels are considered to be high, additional dosimeters should be worn on the extremities.

CHAPTER 4

Basic Radiobiology

Chapter at a glance

It is well known that radiation can cause biologic damage as derived from both animal and human studies. In diagnostic radiology, the benefits associated with radiation exposure far outweigh any risks to the patient. These radiation risks (bioeffects) have received increasing attention since patients received more radiation from diagnostic x-ray examinations than from any other source of radiation exposure (Chapter 3).

The purpose of this chapter is to review the fundamental concepts relating to the manifestation of biologic damage and to describe the early and late effects of radiation exposure. Specifically, radiobiology will be defined and sources of data on the bioeffects of radiation will be identified. This section will be followed by a description of radio sensitivity, dose response models, effects of radiation on cells and water, direct and indirect action of radiation, and the target theory. Finally, the chapter will conclude with a summary of the early and late effects of radiation.

It is essential that technologists have a firm understanding of these topics because:

- Current radiation protection standards and recommendations are based on biologic effects.
- The dose delivered to the patient in radiology can vary from low, to moderate-to-high, depending on the type of examination.
- Dose-response models used in diagnostic radiology suggest that there is no risk-free dose of radiation.

WHAT IS RADIOBIOLOGY?

Radiation transfers energy to biologic systems. The energy is absorbed and subsequently produces a sequence of events leading to biologic expression of harm.

- *Radiobiology* is the study of effects of radiation on biologic systems.

The effects occur at the:

- Molecular level and include physical processes such as ionization and excitation of atoms, and chemical interactions such as the production and reaction of free radicals.
- Cellular level, where damage to DNA and chromosomes occur, leading to damage at the tissue and organ levels (e.g., atrophy).
- Whole-body levels, where the responses are categorized as early and late effects.

This chapter reviews the mechanisms leading to these effects.

ESSENTIAL PHYSICS AND CHEMISTRY

Biologic systems are made up of atoms. The interaction of radiation with a living system requires an understanding of a number of topics in physics and chemistry.

Basic Physics

The physics topics that are of relevance to radiobiology and are of importance to technologists in diagnostic radiology include atomic structure, the nature and properties of x-rays, ionization, excitation, linear energy transfer (LET), and relative biologic effectiveness (RBE).

It is not within the scope of this text to describe any of these in detail; the student must refer to radiological physics textbooks for elaboration. The following points, however, are noteworthy:

- The atom consists of a nucleus positioned at the center of electrons, which occupy specific orbits around the nucleus. Electrons close to the nucleus are tightly bound, and electrons far away from the nucleus are loosely bound and can easily be removed from the atom (ionization).

- The nature of x-rays in terms of production and interaction with matter was the subject of Chapter 2. Essentially, x-rays can produce ionization and excitation of atoms in biologic systems.

- *Ionization* is the removal of an electron from an atom. Ionization results in ion pairs, the electron that has been removed and the positively charged atom remaining. Outer-shell electrons are easily removed from the atom since they are loosely bound to the nucleus.

- *Excitation* is a process by which electrons are transferred into orbital levels farther away from the nucleus as a result of energy absorption. Electrons are not removed from the atom.

- Both ionization and excitation can lead to bioeffects. However, the mechanism of excitation is not fully understood.

- *Linear Energy Transfer* (LET) is the efficiency of radiation to produce ionization and excitation. Specifically, LET measures the rate at which energy is transferred from the radiation to the living system. The units of LET are kilo-electron volt per micrometer of length in soft tissue.As LET increases, biologic damage increases. The LET for x-rays used in radiology is approximately 3.0 keV/μm; for alpha particles, the value is 300 keV/μm.

■ *Relative Biologic Effectiveness* (RBE) is the efficiency with which different types of radiation can cause damage to biologic systems. Specifically, the RBE is a ratio of a standard (200 to 250 kVp x-rays) radiation dose required to produce a given biologic effect to the test radiation dose required to produce the same effect. The RBE for diagnostic x-rays is 1.0. As LET increases, RBE increases since high LET produces more ionization compared with low LET radiation.

Basic Chemistry

In diagnostic radiology, most of the interactions of radiation and the patient occur with water, since the body contains from 70% to 85% water. This interaction results in ionization of water, forming ion pairs and free radicals.

■ Radiolysis of water refers to the breakdown of water by radiation leading to chemical reactions as follows:

❑ $H_2O + radiation \rightarrow H_2O^+ + e^-$

❑ $e^- + H_2O \rightarrow H_2O^-$

■ Two ions (H_2O^+ and H_2O^-) are the by-products of the initial interaction.

■ Each of these two ions is unstable and exists for only a short time. Each will dissociate as follows:

❑ $H_2O^+ \rightarrow H^+ + OH^\bullet$

❑ $H_2O^- \rightarrow H^\bullet + OH^-$

■ Now, there are two ions: a hydrogen ion (H^+) and a hydroxyl ion (OH^-); and two free radicals: a hydroxyl free radical ($OH^\bullet$) and a hydrogen free radical ($H^\bullet$).

■ A free radical symbolized by a dot (•), as shown in the above reactions, is an atom or a molecule with an unpaired electron in the outermost orbit.

■ Free radicals are highly unstable chemical species and can react to form other chemical species that are harmful to the cell.

- Two ions, H^+ and OH^- can recombine as follows:
  - ❑ $H^+ + OH^- \rightarrow H_2O$
- Free radicals can also recombine as follows:
  - ❑ $H^\bullet + OH^\bullet \rightarrow H_2O$
- In the last two cases, water is formed and there is no damage to the cell. However, free radicals can react as follows to form other molecules that are toxic to the cell:
  - ❑ $OH^\bullet + OH^\bullet \rightarrow H_2O_2$
  - ❑ $H^\bullet + O_2 \rightarrow HO_2^\bullet$
- H_2O_2 is hydrogen peroxide, which is toxic to the cell.
- $HO_2^\bullet$ is hydroperoxyl free radical, which is highly reactive and can be combined with biologic macromolecules to produce more and more free radicals.

FUNDAMENTAL CONCEPTS OF RADIOBIOLOGY

There are several concepts of radiobiology that are important to the technologist and that provide a foundation for a good understanding of the bioeffects of radiation.

Types of Bioeffects

Bioeffects can be stochastic or deterministic:

- *Stochastic effects* are those for which the probability of occurrence increases with dose and for which there is no threshold dose. Any dose of radiation, however small, has the potential to cause biologic harm. There is no risk-free dose.
- *Deterministic effects* are those for which the severity of the effect increases with increasing dose and for which there is a threshold dose.

Bioeffects can also be somatic effects and genetic effects:

- *Somatic effects* are those that occur in the individual exposed to the radiation.
- *Genetic effects* are hereditary effects and occur in the offspring of the individual exposed to radiation.

Additionally, bioeffects can be discussed as early and late effects.

- *Early effects* appear minutes, hours, days, weeks, or months after exposure to high doses of radiation. Early effects are deterministic effects.

■ *Late effects* occur years after exposure to low doses of radiation. Late effects are stochastic effects.

Early and late effects of radiation will be reviewed further in a later section of this chapter.

Radiosensitivity

The radiation quantity (effective dose) takes into consideration the sensitivity of tissues to radiation exposure. This sensitivity is referred to as radiosensitivity. In 1906, Bergonie and Tribondeau, two French scientists, performed experiments to demonstrate this radiosensitivity of various tissues. Their results generated the law of Bergonie and Tribondeau, which indicates the following:

■ Immature cells (stem cells) are more radiosensitive than mature cells (end cells).

■ Radiosensitivity is directly proportional to the proliferation rate for cells and the growth rate for tissues. As both rates increase, radiosensitivity increases.

■ Young tissues and organs are more radiosensitive than older tissues and organs.

As noted by Bushong, this law "serves to remind us that the fetus is considerably more sensitive to radiation exposure than the child or the mature adult" (1997).

Radiosensitivity also varies with the phases of the cell cycle as follows:

■ The most radiosensitive phase is mitosis (M), which includes prophase, metaphase, anaphase, and telophase.

■ G_2-phase (post-DNA synthesis) is also extremely sensitive.

■ The most radioresistant phase is the S-phase (DNA-synthesis phase).

Certain cell types are more radiosensitive than are others. For example,

■ Lymphocytes, spermatogonia erythroblast, and the crypt cells of the gastrointestinal tract are extremely radiosensitive.

■ Endothelial cells, osteoblasts, and fibroblasts, for example, have moderate radiosensitivity.

■ Muscle cells and nerve cells have low radiosensitivity.

Radiosensitivity for tissues and organs is as follows:

- Lymphoid tissue, bone marrow, and the gonads have a high level of radiosensitivity.
- The skin, gastrointestinal tract, cornea, growing bone, kidney, liver, and thyroid are moderately radiosensitive.
- Muscle, brain tissue, and the spinal cord have a low level of radiosensitivity.

Dose-Response Relationships

A dose-response relationship shows the relationship between a biologic response (bioeffect) as a function of radiation dose. Two popular linear relationships include:

- Linear dose-response relationship without a threshold. This relationship shows that as the dose increases, the biologic response increases. This relationship also indicates that there is no risk-free dose (i.e., no dose of radiation is considered safe).
- Linear dose-response relationship with a threshold. This relationship shows that there is a level of dose—the threshold dose (D_T)—below which no response is observed. At the threshold dose, a response is observed and it (the response) increases as the dose is increased.

Radiation protection standards and guidelines in diagnostic radiology are based on the linear dose-response relationship without a threshold.

Radiation Effects on DNA and Chromosomes

The human cell consists of two major components: the central nucleus surrounded by the cytoplasm.

Target Molecule

Compared with the cytoplasm, the nucleus is more radiosensitive because:

- The nucleus contains target molecules that are essential for cell survival.
- The target molecule is DNA and it is present in all genetic and somatic cells in relatively few numbers.
- DNA is a critical target molecule for radiation.

- Experiments have shown that lower doses of radiation can cause the cell to die when the nucleus (rather than the cytoplasm) is irradiated.

Target Theory

The target theory states that inactivation of the critical target molecule (DNA) after irradiation will cause the cell to die.

Direct and Indirect Effect

Radiation interaction with a cell can be by either direct or indirect action.

- Direct action occurs when the radiation interacts directly with the critical target to cause a series of events (e.g., ionization) leading to changes that are damaging to the cell.
- Indirect action occurs when radiation interacts with other molecules leading to free radicals, which subsequently interact with the critical target molecule to deactivate it.

DNA Damage

DNA is made up of two strands forming a double helix composed of sugar base pairs of adenine, guanine, cytosine, and thiamine. Irradiation of DNA can result in the following events:

- Single-strand breaks or double-strand breaks.
- Both breaks can be repaired.
- Single-strand breaks are less damaging than double-strand breaks, which can lead to cell death.
- Loss or change of base that leads to genetic mutations.
- Interstrand crosslink resulting in a separation of bases.

The previously mentioned lesions produced in DNA by irradiation result in cell death, malignant disease, and genetic effects.

Chromosome Damage

Chromosomes contain DNA, and damage to DNA leads to chromosome damage. Chromosome damage is also referred to as chromosome aberrations (or breaks). These aberrations can be:

- Single-hit aberrations, which can occur via the direct or indirect effect. The hit, which is an interaction of radiation with the chromosome, will cause a noticeable derangement of the chromosome. Examples of single-hit aberrations include chromatid breaks and chromosome deletions.

■ Multi-hit aberrations, which result in dicentrics, ring chromosomes, multicentrics, and reciprocal translocations.

Experiments have demonstrated that these chromosome aberrations lead to malignancies such as Burkitt's lymphoma, acute promyelocytic leukemia, and ovarian cancer. Chromosome deletions, specifically, lead to small cell lung cancer, neuroblastoma, retinoblastoma, and Wilms' tumor.

DETERMINISTIC EFFECTS (EARLY EFFECTS OF RADIATION)

When the whole body is exposed to high doses of radiation (greater than 1 Gy), several bioeffects are observed, depending on the dose. These effects are called early effects since they can occur within minutes, hours, days, weeks, and months after the exposure.

■ Early effects of radiation are considered deterministic effects because the severity of the effect depends on the dose. These effects have a threshold dose and increase with increasing dose.

■ Death is the major effect of whole-body exposure to high doses of radiation.

LD$_{50/60}$

The dose required to kill 50% of the human population in 60 days is termed the lethal dose 50/60 (LD$_{50/60}$). For humans the LD$_{50/60}$ is 3.5 Gy (350 rad).

Acute Radiation Syndromes

Exposure to large doses of radiation to the whole body will result in the following syndromes:

■ *Bone marrow syndrome.* This syndrome occurs after an acute whole-body exposure of 2 to 10 Gy. The dose affects the stem cells in the bone marrow and other blood-forming organs.

■ *Gastrointestinal syndrome.* This syndrome occurs after an acute whole-body exposure of doses between 10 and

100 Gy. Damage to the crypt cells of the small intestines will cause death, which occurs much faster than that caused by the bone marrow syndrome.

■ *Central nervous system (CNS) syndrome.* This syndrome is also referred to as the cerebrovascular syndrome and requires doses in excess of 100 Gy. Death results because blood vessels in the brain are damaged, leading to edema that causes an increase in skull pressure.

Early or deterministic effects can occur in local tissues, such as the skin and gonads, the hemopoietic system, and cell chromosomes.

■ Damages to the skin include skin erythema (reddening) and epilation (loss of hair), which is a result of damage to the basal cells of the epidermis.

■ The principal effect of high doses of radiation on the gonads (ovaries and testes) is atrophy (reduction in size). In women, the oocyte is highly radiosensitive. Radiation exposure of the ovaries can delay or suppress menstruation, as well as cause temporary or permanent sterility. A dose of 2 Gy will cause temporary sterility; 5 Gy will cause permanent sterility.

■ In men, the spermatogonia are most radiosensitive compared with spermatocytes and spermatids. A dose of 100 mGy decreases the spermatozoa count. A dose of 2 Gy produces temporary sterility; 5 Gy will produce permanent sterility. Spermatogonia are also considered to be among the most radiosensitive of body cells (as well as lymphocytes).

■ The blood system or hemopoietic system is made up of the bone marrow, lymphoid tissue, and circulating blood. The main effect of radiation on this system is to reduce the number of blood cells in the peripheral circulation. Among the blood cells, lymphocytes are the most radiosensitive.

■ Chromosomal damage includes single- and multiple-chromatid breaks, ring chromosomes, and dicentrics, as well as reciprocal translocations.